FELICIA K

Senior Fitness at Home: Embracing Your Golden Years with Grace and Vitality

A Senior's Guide to Staying Strong and Agile

Copyright © 2024 by Felicia K

All rights reserved. No part of this publication may be reproduced, stored or transmitted in any form or by any means, electronic, mechanical, photocopying, recording, scanning, or otherwise without written permission from the publisher. It is illegal to copy this book, post it to a website, or distribute it by any other means without permission.

Disclaimer

The exercises and advice in this book are intended as a guide to fitness and are not tailored to the individual reader. Before beginning any new exercise program, it is recommended that you consult with your physician or other healthcare provider.

The author and publisher of this book are not healthcare professionals. The information provided in this book is based on the author's experiences and the latest research at the time of publication. However, it should not be considered as medical or professional advice.

Neither the author nor the publisher of this book shall be liable for any physical, emotional, or financial damages that might occur due to following the exercises or advice contained in this book. Readers are encouraged to exercise caution and not exceed their limits while performing the exercises described in this book.

Remember, safety first: always use proper form and technique, and never force or strain. Individual results may vary, and the effectiveness of any exercise program will depend on each individual's physical condition.

Using this book, you acknowledge and agree to do so at your own risk.

First edition

This book was professionally typeset on Reedsy.
Find out more at reedsy.com

Contents

1

INTRODUCTION

Welcome to a health, vitality, and empowerment journey in your senior years! As we age, the role of fitness in maintaining our quality of life becomes increasingly significant. This book, "Senior Fitness at Home," is a dedicated guide to help you stay strong, agile, and healthy from home.

Understanding the Importance of Fitness in Your Senior Years

Fitness is not just about physical well-being; it's a gateway to a fuller, more vibrant life. As seniors, staying active is crucial for various reasons. It helps manage and prevent chronic illnesses, maintain independence, improve mental health, and enhance overall quality of life. Regular exercise can boost your energy, maintain your independence, and manage symptoms of illness or pain. Even more importantly, it can improve your mood and overall well-being.

How to Use This Book

"Senior Fitness at Home" is structured to be your companion in creating a personalized fitness routine that resonates with your lifestyle and physical capabilities. Each chapter in this book addresses a key aspect of senior fitness - from strength training and cardiovascular health to nutrition and mental well-being. We provide practical advice, easy-to-follow exercises, and tips to make your fitness journey enjoyable and effective.

- Step-by-Step Guides: You'll find detailed instructions for exercises tailored to senior fitness levels. These include illustrations and modifications to suit various needs and abilities.
- Realistic Advice: This book offers practical tips for overcoming common challenges, such as joint pain or limited mobility, and how to execute exercises safely.
- Inspirational Stories: To keep you motivated, we've included stories from other seniors who have successfully incorporated fitness into their lives.

Setting Realistic Fitness Goals

Setting realistic goals is a key component of your fitness journey. It's important to acknowledge that everyone's body is different, and what works for one person may not work for another. This book will guide you in setting achievable goals based on your fitness level, health conditions, and personal preferences. We encourage a gradual approach – starting slow, celebrating small victories, and progressively building up your routine.

Remember, the goal of this book is not just to help you stay fit; it's to empower you to live your senior years with zest and independence. Whether you're looking to strengthen your muscles, improve your balance, or stay active, "Senior Fitness at Home" guides you every step of the way. Let's embark on this rewarding journey together!

2

Chapter 1: Evaluating Your Current Fitness Level

efore embarking on any new fitness regimen, seniors must evaluate their current fitness level. This evaluation is the foundation for creating a safe and effective exercise program tailored to individual needs. A vital first step in this process is consulting with a healthcare professional, such as your doctor, to ensure the planned activities are appropriate for your health status and physical capabilities. This chapter will guide you through assessing your health and physical capabilities and tailoring exercises to meet your unique needs. By taking these steps, you can confidently embark on your fitness journey, knowing that your regimen aligns with your health requirements and goals.

Assessing Your Health and Physical Capabilities

The first step in your fitness journey is assessing your health and physical capabilities. This self-assessment helps understand your starting point and set realistic fitness goals.

- Self-Evaluation: Start by asking yourself some basic questions about your current activity levels and any physical limitations. How often are you currently active? Are there any exercises you find difficult? Do you experience pain during certain activities?
- Basic Fitness Tests: Simple tests can be done at home to assess your balance, flexibility, strength, and endurance. For instance, time how long you can hold a balance pose or count how many sit-to-stand exercises you can do in a minute.
- Monitor Your Vital Signs: Pay attention to your heart rate, blood pressure, and breathing during physical activity. These indicators can provide valuable information about your cardiovascular and overall health.

Consulting with Healthcare Professionals

Before starting any new exercise program, consulting with healthcare professionals is crucial. This is especially important if you have any pre-existing health conditions or concerns.

- Medical Clearance: A check-up with your doctor can ensure that it's safe for you to increase your physical activity. Discuss any concerns you have, such as heart health or joint pain.
- Specialist Advice: In some cases, you might benefit from consulting specialists such as a physiotherapist, a cardiologist, or an orthopedist. They can provide specific advice and precautions based on your health status.
- Medication Review: If you are on any medications, review them with your doctor. Some medicines can affect your heart rate and overall response to exercise.

Tailoring Exercises to Your Individual Needs

Once you understand your current fitness level and have consulted with healthcare professionals, the next step is to tailor exercises to your needs.

- Personalized Exercise Plan: Based on your assessment and consultations, develop an exercise plan that caters to your unique needs and goals. Consider factors like endurance, strength, flexibility, and balance.
- Start Slowly: If you're new to exercising or getting back into it after a break, start slowly. Gradually increase the intensity and duration of your workouts.
- Adapt and Modify: Be prepared to adapt and modify exercises as needed. Listen to your body and adjust your routine to your feelings during and after workouts.
- Incorporate Variety: To make your exercise routine well-rounded, include various activities. This addresses different aspects of fitness and keeps the routine interesting and engaging.

By carefully evaluating your fitness level and working with healthcare professionals, you can create a safe and effective exercise plan tailored to your unique needs. This thoughtful approach ensures that your journey to improved health and fitness is enjoyable and beneficial.

3

Chapter 2: Essentials of a Senior-Friendly Home Gym

Creating a senior-friendly home gym is about designing a safe, comfortable space with the right tools to meet your fitness needs. This chapter will guide you through setting up your home gym, focusing on the basics of equipment, creating a safe workout space, and adapting your home for injury prevention.

Equipment Basics: What You Need

Simplicity and functionality are key in equipment for a senior-friendly home gym. You don't need a lot of expensive or bulky equipment to get a good workout.

Here are some essentials:

- **Resistance Bands: These are versatile, easy to store, and perfect for various exercises to improve strength and flexibility.**
- **Dumbbells or Hand Weights: Light to moderate weights can be**

used for strength training. Opt for weights with a comfortable grip.

- **Stability Ball: Great for balance and core strengthening exercises. Ensure you choose the right size for your height.**
- **Yoga Mat: Provides cushioning and grip for floor exercises, yoga, and stretching.**
- **Chair or Bench: A sturdy chair or bench is essential for seated exercises or as support for balance exercises.**

Creating a Safe Workout Space

The space where you exercise should be safe and conducive to your workout routine.

Consider the following:

- Sufficient Space: Ensure there's enough room to move freely without the risk of bumping into furniture or other objects.
- Good Lighting: A well-lit area reduces the risk of falls and helps you see clearly while exercising.
- Non-Slip Surface: Secure rugs or carpets with non-slip pads or opt for a non-slip flooring surface to prevent slips and falls.
- Ventilation: Good air circulation is important, especially during physical exertion. Ensure your workout area is well-ventilated.

Adapting Your Home for Injury Prevention

Preventing injuries is paramount, especially for seniors engaging in physical activity. Here are some adaptations you can make:

- Clear Pathways: Keep the path to and around your workout area clear of clutter to prevent trips and falls.
- Safety Equipment: Install grab bars or railings where necessary, especially where balance exercises will be performed.
- Emergency Plan: Have a phone accessible in case of emergencies. It's also wise to let someone know when you're about to exercise.
- Regular Equipment Checks: Regularly inspect your exercise equipment for wear and tear to ensure it remains safe.
- Setting up a senior-friendly home gym doesn't have to be complicated or expensive. With the right equipment, a safe space, and a few adaptations, you can create an effective and enjoyable workout area in your home. This environment will support your physical health and provide a sense of independence and confidence in your fitness journey.

Essentials of a Senior-Friendly Home Gym

Creating a senior-friendly home gym is about designing a safe, comfortable space with the right tools to meet your fitness needs. This chapter will guide you through setting up your home gym, focusing on the basics of equipment, creating a safe workout space, and adapting your home for injury prevention.

Equipment Basics: What You Need

Simplicity and functionality are key in equipment for a senior-friendly home gym. You don't need a lot of expensive or bulky equipment to get a good workout. Here are some essentials:

- Resistance Bands: These are versatile, easy to store, and perfect for various exercises to improve strength and flexibility.
- Dumbbells or Hand Weights: Light to moderate weights can be used for strength training. Opt for weights with a comfortable grip.
- Stability Ball: Great for balance and core strengthening exercises. Ensure you choose the right size for your height.
- Yoga Mat: Provides cushioning and grip for floor exercises, yoga, and stretching.
- Chair or Bench: A sturdy chair or bench is essential for seated exercises or as support for balance exercises.

Creating a Safe Workout Space

The space where you exercise should be safe and conducive to your workout routine. Consider the following:

- Sufficient Space: Ensure there's enough room to move freely without the risk of bumping into furniture or other objects.
- Good Lighting: A well-lit area reduces the risk of falls and helps you see clearly while exercising.
- Non-Slip Surface: Secure rugs or carpets with non-slip pads or opt for a non-slip flooring surface to prevent slips and falls.
- Ventilation: Good air circulation is important, especially during physical exertion. Ensure your workout area is well-ventilated.

Adapting Your Home for Injury Prevention

Preventing injuries is paramount, especially for seniors engaging in physical activity. Here are some adaptations you can make:

- Clear Pathways: Keep the path to and around your workout area clear of clutter to prevent trips and falls.
- Safety Equipment: Install grab bars or railings where necessary, especially where balance exercises will be performed.
- Emergency Plan: Have a phone accessible in case of emergencies. It's also wise to let someone know when you're about to exercise.
- Regular Equipment Checks: Regularly inspect your exercise equipment for wear and tear to ensure it remains safe.

Setting up a senior-friendly home gym doesn't have to be complicated or expensive. With the right equipment, a safe space, and a few adaptations, you can create an effective and enjoyable workout area in your home. This environment will support your physical health and provide a sense of independence and confidence in your fitness journey.

4

Chapter 3: Strength Training for Seniors

Strength training is a vital component of a senior's fitness regimen, offering numerous benefits for health and well-being. This chapter delves into the advantages of strength training, highlights safe and effective exercises, and guides building a routine from beginner to advanced levels.

Benefits of Strength Training

As we age, we lose muscle mass and strength, a process known as sarcopenia. Strength training combats this decline, offering several key benefits:

- Increased Muscle Mass and Strength: Regular strength training helps maintain and increase muscle mass and strength, which is essential for everyday activities.
- Improved Bone Density: It reduces the risk of osteoporosis by stressing and thus strengthening the bones.
- Enhanced Balance and Coordination: This reduces the risk of falls,

a major concern for seniors.

- Better Joint Flexibility: Strength training helps maintain joint flexibility, reducing arthritis symptoms and other joint issues.
- Boosted Metabolic Rate: Building muscle helps increase the resting metabolic rate, aiding in weight management.
- Enhanced Mental Health: It can improve mood, boost self-confidence, and has been shown to reduce symptoms of depression and anxiety.

Safe and Effective Strength Exercises

When it comes to strength training, safety is paramount. Here are some effective exercises that are generally safe for seniors:

- Wall Push-Ups: A gentler alternative to traditional push-ups, focusing on upper body strength.
- Chair Squats: These strengthen the legs and core while using a chair for support.
- Bicep Curls: Can be done with light dumbbells or resistance bands to strengthen the arms.
- Leg Lifts: Great for strengthening the thighs and improving balance.
- Seated Rows: Using a resistance band, this exercise is excellent for back and arm strength.

Always start with light weights or low resistance and focus on slow, controlled movements. It's important to breathe properly during these exercises — exhale during the exertion phase and inhale during the relaxation phase.

Building a Routine: From Beginners to Advanced

When starting, it's crucial to build your strength training routine gradually:

- Beginner: Focus on learning the correct form and getting accustomed to the exercises. Start with lighter weights and fewer repetitions.
- Intermediate: As you grow stronger, gradually increase the weight or resistance and add more repetitions.
- Advanced: Once you're comfortable, incorporate more challenging exercises or combinations, and increase the frequency of your workouts.

It's important to listen to your body and not push too hard. Rest is crucial in any strength training regimen, allowing muscles to recover and grow stronger. Aim for two to three strength training sessions weekly, ensuring you rest each muscle group for at least a day before exercising again.

Remember, it's always recommended to consult with a healthcare provider before starting any new exercise routine, especially if you have pre-existing health conditions. By incorporating regular strength training into your lifestyle, you can significantly enhance your quality of life in your senior years.

5

Chapter 5: Cardiovascular Health and Endurance

Cardiovascular health is crucial for seniors, as it greatly impacts overall well-being and functional independence. This chapter focuses on heart health for seniors, suggests low-impact cardio exercises suitable for home environments, and discusses how to balance cardio with other types of exercise.

Heart Health for Seniors

As we age, our heart and blood vessels change, making heart health an important focus for seniors. Regular cardiovascular exercise can offer significant benefits:

- Improving Heart Efficiency: Cardio exercises strengthen the heart muscle, improving its ability to pump blood more efficiently.
- Reducing Risk of Heart Disease: Active seniors often have a lower risk of developing heart conditions.
- Controlling Blood Pressure: Regular cardio exercise can help

manage high blood pressure.

- Improving Cholesterol Levels: It helps balance good (HDL) and bad (LDL) cholesterol.
- Boosting Circulation and Oxygen Delivery: Enhanced circulation promotes better oxygen and nutrient delivery throughout the body.

Low-Impact Cardio Exercises You Can Do at Home

Low-impact exercises are particularly suitable for seniors as they are less stressful on the joints. Here are some effective cardio exercises that can be easily done at home:

- Walking: Brisk walking indoors or on a treadmill, if space allows, is excellent for cardiovascular health.
- Step Exercises: Using a low step or stair, step exercises can increase your heart rate without high impact.
- Seated Aerobics: These are great for those with mobility issues, involving movements that raise the heart rate while sitting.
- Dance: Dancing to your favorite music is fun and an excellent way to improve cardiovascular health.
- Cycling: A stationary bike provides a good cardio workout with minimal joint stress.

It's important to start slowly and gradually increasing your workout duration and intensity. Aim for at least 150 minutes of moderate-intensity aerobic activity per week, as recommended by health authorities.

Balancing Cardio with Other Types of Exercise

While cardio is important, it's just one component of a well-rounded fitness regimen. It should be balanced with other forms of exercise:

- Strength Training: As mentioned earlier, strength training is vital for muscle and bone health.
- Flexibility Exercises: Activities like stretching or yoga help maintain joint range of motion and prevent injuries.
- Balance Training: Exercises that enhance balance can reduce the risk of falls, a common concern for seniors.

A balanced routine incorporating all these elements can maximize health benefits and reduce the risks of overuse injuries. It's also important to include rest days to allow your body to recover.

Always listen to your body and adjust your exercise routine as needed. Regular physical activity, tailored to your abilities and health status, can significantly enhance your cardiovascular health and overall quality of life as you age.

6

Chapter 6: Flexibility and Balance

Flexibility and balance are crucial components of a senior's fitness routine, significantly supporting overall mobility and fall prevention. This chapter explores the importance of flexibility and balance in preventing falls, provides examples of stretching and balance exercises, and discusses the integration of yoga and tai chi principles.

The Importance of Flexibility and Balance in Preventing Falls

Our muscles lose strength and elasticity as we age, and our joints may become less flexible. This can lead to a decrease in balance and coordination, increasing the risk of falls. Improving flexibility and balance is key to preventing falls, which are a major cause of injury among seniors.

- Flexibility: Enhanced flexibility improves the range of motion in your joints, reduces stiffness, and helps you easily perform daily activities.

- Balance: Good balance helps maintain stability and body posture, which is essential for preventing falls and maintaining independence.

Stretching and Balance Exercises

There are many exercises that seniors can do to improve flexibility and balance. Some effective ones include:

- Toe Stands: This simple exercise improves balance and strengthens the legs. Stand behind a chair for support, slowly stand on tiptoes, hold, and then lower.
- Leg Lifts: Stand behind a chair, lift one leg to the side, and hold and lower. This enhances balance and leg strength.
- Shoulder Stretch: Helps improve upper body flexibility. Reach one arm across your body and lightly press it towards your chest.
- Neck Stretch: Gently turn your head from side to side and tilt it towards your shoulder to stretch your neck muscles.
- Hamstring Stretch: Sitting on the edge of a chair, extend one leg in front, and lean forward gently, keeping your back straight.

It's important to perform these exercises in a safe environment and to avoid any movements that cause pain.

Incorporating Yoga and Tai Chi Principles

Yoga and Tai Chi are excellent for seniors as they combine flexibility, balance, and mindfulness.

- Yoga: It involves various poses that enhance flexibility and balance. Many yoga poses can be modified and done with the support of a chair or against a wall for safety.
- Tai Chi: This form of gentle martial arts focuses on slow, deliberate movements and deep breathing. Tai Chi enhances balance, flexibility, and mental focus.

Both practices improve physical aspects and offer mental health benefits, such as reduced stress and improved concentration.

Incorporating flexibility and balance exercises into your daily routine can significantly enhance your quality of life in your senior years. These practices reduce the risk of falls, promote independence, and contribute to overall physical and mental well-being. Always consult a healthcare provider before starting any new exercise regimen, especially if you have existing health conditions.

7

Chapter 7: Nutrition for Senior Fitness

Nutrition plays a pivotal role in the health and fitness of seniors. As the body ages, its nutritional needs evolve, necessitating adjustments in diet to maintain energy, muscle health, and overall well-being. This chapter covers the specific nutritional needs of older adults, how to eat for energy and muscle health, and the importance of hydration, particularly concerning exercise.

Nutritional Needs for Older Adults

The dietary requirements of seniors differ from those of younger adults due to changes in metabolism, digestive system efficiency, and nutrient absorption. Key aspects include:

- Reduced Caloric Needs: As metabolism slows with age, seniors typically require fewer calories. However, the need for nutrients remains high, emphasizing the importance of nutrient-dense foods.
- Protein: Adequate protein intake is crucial for preserving muscle

mass and strength. Sources like lean meats, fish, eggs, dairy products, legumes, and nuts should be included in the diet.

- Calcium and Vitamin D: Essential for bone health, these can be sourced from dairy products, fortified foods, and appropriate sun exposure.
- Fiber: Important for digestive health, fiber can be found in fruits, vegetables, whole grains, and legumes.
- B Vitamins: Particularly vitamin B12, which is vital for maintaining nerve function and blood cells, can become harder to absorb with age. Fortified cereals, lean meats, and some seafood can help meet this need.

Eating for Energy and Muscle Health

Maintaining energy levels and muscle health is essential for an active lifestyle:

- Balanced Meals: Include a variety of foods in your diet – fruits, vegetables, whole grains, lean protein, and healthy fats.
- Regular, Small Meals: Smaller, more frequent meals can effectively manage seniors' energy levels and metabolism.
- Lean Protein: Incorporate lean protein into each meal to support muscle repair and growth, especially important after exercising.

Hydration and its Importance in Exercise

Hydration is a critical, yet often overlooked, aspect of senior fitness:

- Water Intake: With age, the body's sense of thirst diminishes, increasing the risk of dehydration. It's important to drink water regularly, not just when thirsty.

- During Exercise: Hydration is important to replace fluids lost through sweating and maintain circulatory function and muscle health.
- Signs of Dehydration: Be aware of dehydration signs, such as dry mouth, fatigue, dizziness, and dark-colored urine.

Good nutrition and adequate hydration are the foundations of a healthy, active lifestyle for seniors. By understanding and addressing their specific dietary needs, older adults can significantly enhance their fitness, energy levels, and overall quality of life. As always, it's advisable to consult with a healthcare provider or a dietitian to tailor dietary choices to individual health needs and fitness goals.

8

Chapter 8: Mental Health and Exercise

Exercise is not just a physical activity; it also plays a significant role in maintaining and enhancing mental health, especially for seniors. This chapter explores how exercise can be a powerful tool for cognitive health, its impact on stress reduction and mental well-being, and the benefits of mind-body exercises.

Exercise as a Tool for Cognitive Health

Regular physical activity has a direct impact on brain health. For seniors, this can translate into various cognitive benefits:

- Improved Memory and Brain Function: Exercise increases heart rate, promoting blood and oxygen flow to the brain, and improving memory and cognitive functions.
- Neuroprotection: Physical activity can stimulate the production of chemicals in the brain that affect the health of brain cells and the growth of new blood vessels in the brain.
- Delaying the Onset of Cognitive Decline: Regular exercise is

linked with a lower risk of cognitive decline and conditions like Alzheimer's disease and dementia.

Stress Reduction and Mental Well-Being

The mental health benefits of exercise are just as important as the physical ones:

- Reduction in Stress and Anxiety: Physical activity produces endorphins, the brain's natural mood lifters, which can reduce stress and anxiety.
- Enhanced Mood: Regular exercise can improve overall mood, increase self-esteem, and reduce symptoms of depression.
- Improved Sleep: Regular physical activity can help seniors regulate their sleep patterns, leading to better sleep quality.

Mind-Body Exercises and Their Benefits

Mind-body exercises combine physical activity with a focus on mental and emotional well-being. They include practices like yoga, tai chi, and pilates. Benefits of these exercises include:

- Increased Mindfulness: These practices encourage a focus on the present moment, which can reduce stress and promote a state of mental calmness.
- Improved Balance and Flexibility: Mind-body exercises often focus on improving balance and flexibility, which are crucial for seniors.
- Enhanced Body Awareness: Regular practice can lead to a greater awareness of the body, which can help recognize and respond to

stress symptoms more effectively.

Incorporating regular exercise into a senior's routine can be a powerful way to enhance not only physical health but also mental and cognitive well-being. As exercise becomes a regular part of life, seniors may notice an improvement in their overall mood, stress levels, and cognitive functions. Choosing enjoyable and suitable activities for one's physical capabilities is important to ensure consistency and reap the full mental health benefits. Consult with healthcare professionals before starting any new exercise regimen.

9

Chapter 9: Overcoming Common Challenges

Embarking on a fitness journey in your senior year can be rewarding and challenging. Common obstacles such as arthritis and joint pain, managing chronic conditions, and maintaining motivation are often part of the journey. This chapter addresses these challenges, offering strategies for dealing with them effectively.

Dealing with Arthritis and Joint Pain

Arthritis and joint pain are common among seniors and can impede the ability to exercise. However, there are ways to manage these conditions:

- Low-Impact Exercises: Walking, swimming, or cycling can be less stressful on your joints than high-impact exercises.
- Strength Training: Strengthening the muscles around the affected joints can help reduce overall joint stress.
- Flexibility Exercises: Regular stretching can improve joint range of

motion and alleviate stiffness.
- Warm-Up and Cool-Down: Properly warming up before exercising and cooling down afterward can help prevent pain and stiffness.
- Pain Management: Consult with a healthcare provider for advice on pain management, which may include medications, physical therapy, or alternative treatments.

Exercising with Chronic Conditions

Many seniors live with chronic conditions like heart disease, diabetes, or osteoporosis. While these conditions can complicate the exercise process, they don't have to be a barrier:

- Personalized Exercise Plan: Work with healthcare professionals to create an exercise plan that accommodates your condition.
- Monitoring: Keep track of relevant health indicators, such as blood sugar levels or blood pressure, especially before and after exercising.
- Adjusting Intensity and Duration: Start with low-intensity exercises and gradually increase as tolerated. Be mindful of the duration, and don't overexert yourself.
- Being Aware of Symptoms: Recognize the signs and symptoms that indicate you should stop exercising and consult a doctor.

Staying Motivated and Overcoming Plateaus

Maintaining motivation and dealing with plateaus are challenges for exercisers of all ages, but they can be particularly daunting for seniors:

- Set Realistic Goals: Clear, achievable goals can help maintain focus and motivation.

- Variety in Routine: Mixing up your exercise routine can prevent boredom and stimulate different muscle groups.
- Social Support: Joining a group or exercising with friends can increase accountability and make exercising more enjoyable.
- Tracking Progress: Keep a journal or log to track your progress. This can be encouraging, especially during plateaus.
- Celebrating Success: Acknowledge and celebrate your achievements, no matter how small they may seem.

Overcoming these common challenges requires patience, persistence, and a positive attitude. Remember, the fitness journey is personal and unique to each individual. It's about progress, not perfection. By understanding your body's needs and limitations and adapting your approach accordingly, you can enjoy a healthy and active lifestyle in your senior years.

10

Chapter 10: Building a Sustainable Routine

For seniors, building a sustainable and adaptable fitness routine is the key to reaping the long-term benefits of exercise. This chapter focuses on creating a long-term fitness plan, tracking progress and adjusting goals, and maintaining an active and fit lifestyle.

Creating a Long-term Fitness Plan

A long-term fitness plan for seniors should be realistic, flexible, and tailored to individual health conditions and interests. Here's how to create one:

- Assess Your Current Lifestyle: Consider your daily routine, physical abilities, and health issues.
- Set Achievable Goals: Goals should be specific, measurable, attainable, relevant, and time-bound (SMART). They include improving balance, increasing strength, or enhancing flexibility.
- Incorporate Various Exercise Types: Include cardiovascular exer-

cises, strength training, flexibility workouts, and balance activities.

- Plan for Gradual Progression: Start with shorter, less intense workouts, gradually increasing duration and intensity.
- Be Adaptable: Be prepared to modify your plan as your needs and abilities change.

Tracking Progress and Adjusting Goals

Regularly tracking your progress helps you stay motivated and adjust your goals as needed:

- Keep an Exercise Diary: Record your workouts, noting types of exercises, duration, and how you felt during and after each session.
- Monitor Your Health Indicators: Keep track of relevant health metrics, such as blood pressure, weight, or cholesterol levels, as these can indicate your fitness progress.
- Regular Assessments: Every few months, reassess your fitness level to see if you can increase the intensity of your workouts or try new activities.
- Adjust Goals as Needed: Based on your progress, you may need to set or modify new goals.

Staying Active and Fit Through the Years

Maintaining an active lifestyle as you age is essential for overall well-being:

- Consistency is Key: Aim to make exercise a regular part of your daily routine. Consistency is more important than intensity.

- Find Activities You Enjoy: You're more likely to stick with a fitness plan if you enjoy the activities. Experiment with different exercises to find what you like best.
- Stay Socially Engaged: Participate in group classes or activities. Social engagement can be a powerful motivator.
- Listen to Your Body: Pay attention to your body's signals. Rest when needed, and don't push through pain.
- Lifelong Learning: Stay open to learning new exercises or techniques. This not only keeps your routine interesting but can also be beneficial for your cognitive health.

Building a sustainable fitness routine is a continuous process that evolves with your changing needs and abilities. By staying committed, adaptable, and patient with your progress, you can enjoy a healthier, more active lifestyle well into your senior years. Remember, the goal is to add years to your life and life to your years.

11

Bonus: Sample Tracker

Exercise Tracker
Personal Details:

- Name: ____________________________
- Age: ____________________________
- Starting Date: ____________________
- Health Conditions: ________________________
- Physician's Approval (Yes/No): ___________

Weekly Exercise Goals:

- Total Exercise Days per Week: ___
- Total Exercise Time per Week: ___ hours
- Specific Goals (e.g., flexibility, strength, balance): ________________________

Daily Log:
Date
Exercise Type (e.g., Walking, Stretching)
Duration

Intensity (Low/Medium/High)

Notes (e.g., how you felt, any discomfort)

2024-01-30

2024-01-31

2024-02-01

2024-02-02

2024-02-03

2024-02-04

2024-02-05

Weekly Reflection:

- Achievements this week:
- Challenges faced:
- Plans/Adjustments for next week:

Instructions:

1. **Consult a Physician:** Before starting any new exercise routine, getting approval from a healthcare provider is essential, especially if there are existing health conditions.
2. **Set Realistic Goals:** Begin with achievable targets in terms of days per week and duration.
3. **Diversify Exercise Types:** Include a mix of activities focusing on strength, balance, flexibility, and cardiovascular health.
4. **Monitor Intensity:** Ensure the exercise intensity is appropriate - it should be challenging but not overwhelming.
5. **Take Notes:** Document how each exercise session felt, noting any discomfort or achievements.
6. **Reflect Weekly:** At the end of each week, review progress and plan for the following week, adjusting as necessary.

This tracker is a basic model and can be adjusted based on specific exercises recommended for the individual, their health status, and fitness goals.

12

Conclusion

As we conclude "Senior Fitness at Home," reflecting on the journey we've embarked upon is important. This guide aims to educate, inspire, and empower you to take charge of your health and wellness during your senior years. By understanding the multifaceted benefits of fitness - from bolstering physical strength and flexibility to enhancing mental well-being and cognitive health - you can appreciate the profound impact regular exercise can have on your quality of life.

We've explored the importance of tailoring fitness routines to individual needs, recognizing that each person's body and health circumstances are unique. The comprehensive approach of assessing current fitness levels, consulting with healthcare professionals, and gradually building a routine ensures a safe and effective path to fitness. Incorporating strength training, cardiovascular exercises, flexibility, and balance activities, alongside nutrition and mental health considerations, create a well-rounded and holistic approach to senior fitness.

The concept of a senior-friendly home gym, utilizing simple yet effective equipment and creating a safe environment, underscores the idea that fitness is accessible and achievable from the comfort of your home. This demystifies that maintaining fitness in later years is complex or requires expensive resources.

Furthermore, the emphasis on overcoming common challenges like arthritis, joint pain, and staying motivated amidst life's flows speaks to the realistic approach of this guide. It acknowledges seniors' hurdles and provides practical strategies to overcome them, reinforcing that persistence and adaptability are key.

In building a sustainable routine, the focus shifts to the long-term perspective. It's about creating an enjoyable, rewarding, and continually evolving lifestyle change to match your changing needs. By integrating fitness into daily life, not as a chore but as a source of joy and empowerment, you can enhance your physical health and your independence, confidence, and overall sense of fulfillment.

Remember, the fitness journey is not a race; it's a personal journey that values progress over perfection. Whether starting with gentle stretches or building up to more robust exercises, every step you take is towards a healthier, more vibrant life. So, embrace this journey with enthusiasm and patience, and let "Senior Fitness at Home" be your guide to a happier, healthier you in your senior years. The goal is to add years to your life and more importantly, life to your years.

www.ingramcontent.com/pod-product-compliance
Lightning Source LLC
Chambersburg PA
CBHW050753250726
48662CB00005B/2200